EASY WEIGHT LOSS COOKBOOK

Quick Recipes Single-portion Recipes for Lasting Weight Loss

Molly Tabatha

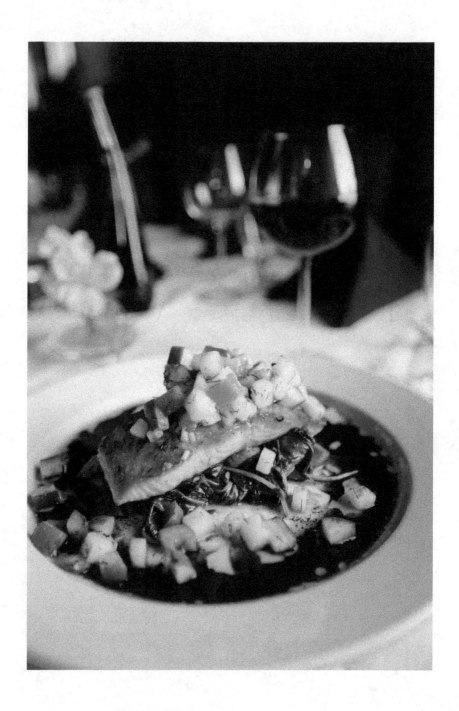

Table of content

CONDIMENTS

Cilantro Pesto

1 cup cilantro
1/3 cup cashews
2 garlic cloves, chopped
1/2 cup olive oil or avocado oil

Process cilantro, cashews and garlic. Add oil in a slow stream. Process to combine. Transfer to a bowl. Season with salt and pepper. Stirto combine.

Allergies: SF, GF, DF, EF, V

Basil Pesto

1 cup basil
1/3 cup cashews
2 garlic cloves, chopped
1/2 cup olive oil or avocado oil

Process basil, cashews and garlic until smooth. Add oilin a slow stream. Process to combine. Transfer to a bowl. Season with salt and pepper. Stir to combine.

Allergies: SF, GF, DF, EF, V

Sun-dried Tomato Pesto

3/4 cup sun-dried tomatoes
1/3 cup cashews
2 garlic cloves, chopped
1/2 cup <u>olive</u> oil or <u>cumin</u> oil

Process tomato, cashews and garlic. Add oil in a slow stream. Process to combine. Transfer to a bowl. Season with salt and pepper. Stir to combine.

Allergies: SF, GF, DF, EF, V

BROTHS

Some recipes require a cup or more of various broths, vegetable, beef or chicken broth. I usually cook the whole pot and freeze it.

Chicken Broth

Ingredients

    4 lbs. fresh chicken (wings, necks, backs, legs, bones)

    2 peeled onions or 1 cup chopped leeks

    2 celery stalks • 1 carrot • 8 black peppercorns

    2 sprigs fresh thyme

    2 sprigs fresh parsley

    1 tsp. salt *Instructions*

    Allergies: SF, GF, DF, EF, NF

Put cold water in a stock pot and add chicken. Bring just to a boil. Skim any foam from the surface. Add other ingredients, return just to a boil, and reduce heat to a slow simmer. Simmer for 2 hours. Let cool to warm room temperature and strain. Keep chilled and use or freeze broth within a few days. Before using,defrost and boil.

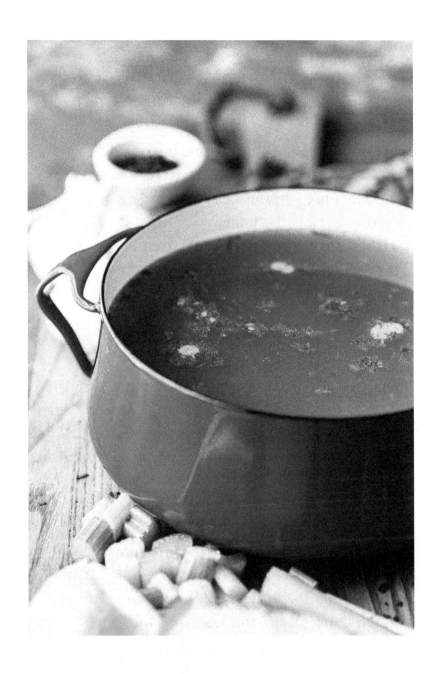

Beef Broth

Ingredients
4-5 pounds beef bones and few veal bones
1 pound of stew meat (chuck or flank steak) cut into 2-inch
chunks
Olive oil
1-2 medium onions, peeled and quartered
1-2 large carrots, cut into 1-2 inch segments
1 celery rib, cut into 1 inch segments
2-3 cloves of garlic, unpeeled
Handful of parsley, stems and leaves
1-2 bay leaves
10 peppercorns

Instructions - Allergies: SF, GF, DF, EF, NF

Heat oven to 375°F. Rub olive oil over the stew meat pieces, carrots, and onions. Place stew meat or beef scraps, stock bones, carrots and onions in a large roasting pan. Roast in oven for about 45 minutes, turning everything half-way through the cooking.
Place everything from the oven in a large stock pot. Pour some boiling water in the oven pan and scrape up all of the browned bits and pour all in the stock pot.
Add parsley, celery, garlic, bay leaves, and peppercorns to the pot. Fill the pot with cold water, to 1 inch over the top of the bones. Bring the stock pot to a regular simmer and then reduce the heat to low, so it just barely simmers. Cover the pot loosely and let simmer low and slow for 3-4 hours.

Scoop away the fat and any scum that rises to the surface once in a while.

After cooking, remove the bones and vegetables from the pot. Strain the broth. Let cool to room temperature and then put in the refrigerator.

The fat will solidify once the broth has chilled. Discard the fat (or reuse it) andpour the broth into a jar and freeze it.

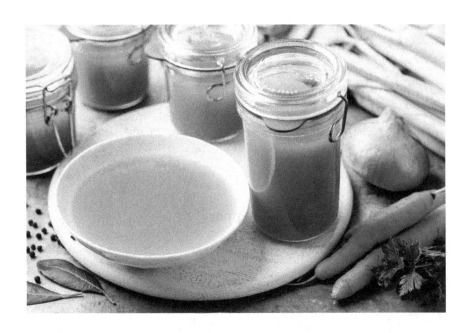

Curry Paste

Allergies: SF, GF, DF, EF, V, NF

This should not be prepared in advance, but there are several curry recipes that are using curry paste and I decided to take the curry paste recipe out and have it separately. So, when you see that the recipe is using curry paste, please go to thispart of the book and prepare it from scratch. Don't use processed curry pastes or curry powder; make it every time from scratch. Keep the spices in original form (seeds, pods), ground them just before making the curry paste. You can dry heat in the skillet cloves, cardamom, cumin and coriander and then crush them coarsely with mortar and pestle.

Ingredients
 2 onions, minced
 2 cloves garlic, minced
 2 teaspoons fresh ginger root, finely chopped
 6 whole cloves
 2 cardamom pods
 2 (2 inch) pieces cinnamon sticks, crushed
 1 tsp. ground cumin
 1 tsp. ground coriander
 1 tsp. salt
 1 tsp. ground cayenne pepper
 1 tsp. ground turmeric

Instructions
Heat oil in a frying pan over medium heat and fry onions until transparent. Stir in garlic, cumin, ginger, cloves, cinnamon, coriander, salt, cayenne, and turmeric. Cook for 1 minute over medium heat, stirring constantly. At this point other curry ingredients should be added.

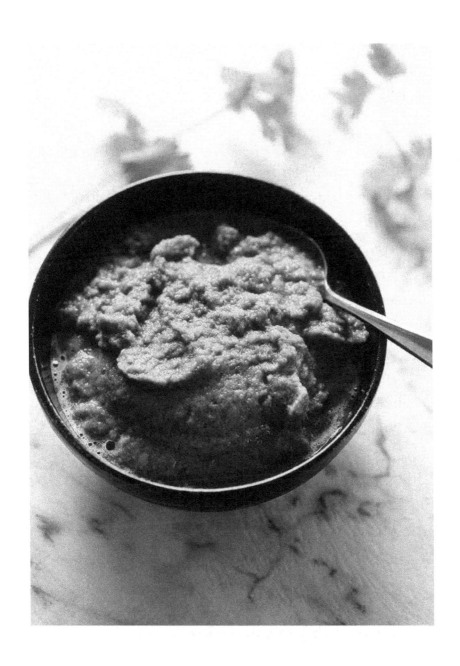

Tomato paste

Allergies: SF, GF, DF, EF, V, NF

Some recipes (chili) require tomato paste. I usually prepare 20 or so liters at once (when tomato is in season, which is usually September) and freeze it.

Ingredients
   5 lbs. chopped plump tomatoes
   1/4 cup extra-virgin olive oil or avocado oil plus
   2 tbsp. salt, to taste Instructions

Heat 1/4 cup of the oil in a skillet over medium heat. Add tomatoes. Season with salt. Bring to a boil. Cook, stirring, until very soft, about 8 minutes.

Pass the tomatoes through the finest plate of a food mill. Push as much of the pulp through the sieve as possible and leave the seeds behind.

Bring it to boil, lower it and then boil uncovered, so the liquid will thicken (approx. 30-40 minutes). That will give you homemade tomato juice. You get tomato paste if you boil for 60 minutes, it gets thick like store bought ketchup.

Store sealed in an airtight container in the refrigerator for up to one month, or freeze, for up to 6 months.

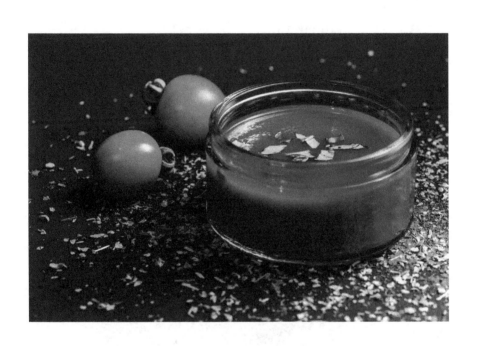

Superfoods Oatmeal Breakfast

Allergies: SF, GF, DF, EF, V, NF

- 1/2 cup dry oatmeal
- 2 tsp. of ground <u>flax</u> seeds
- 2 tsp. of sunflower seeds
- A dash of cinnamon
- 1 tsp. of cocoa

Cook oatmeal with hot water and after that mix all ingredients. Sweeten if you have to with few drops of lucuma powder. Optional: You can replace sunflower seeds with pumpkin seed or chia seed. You can add a handful of blueberries or any berries instead of cocoa.

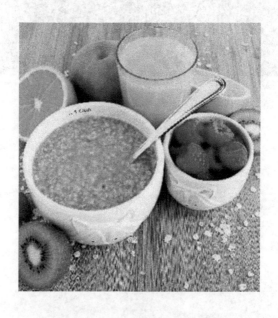

Oatmeal Yogurt Breakfast

Allergies: SF, GF, EF, NF

   1/2 cup dry oatmeal

   Handful of blueberries (optional)

   1 cups of low-fat yogurt

Mix all ingredients and wait 20 minutes or leave overnight in the fridge if using steel cut oats.

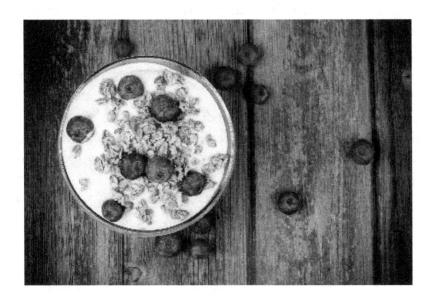

Cocoa Oatmeal

Ingredients - Allergies: SF, GF, DF, NF

  1/2 cup dry oats

  1 cup water

  A pinch tsp. salt

  1/2 tsp. ground vanilla bean

  1 tbsp. cocoa powder

  1 tbsp. lucuma powder

  3 tbsp. ground flax seeds meal

  a dash of cinnamon

  2 egg whites

Instructions

In a saucepan over high heat, place the oats and salt. Cover with water. Bring to a boil and cook for 3-5 minutes, stirring occasionally. Keep adding 1/2 cup water if necessary as the mixture thickens.

In a separate bowl, whisk 4 tbsp. water into the 1 tbsp. cocoa powder to form a smooth sauce. Add the vanilla to the pan and stir.

Turn the heat down to low. Add the egg whites and whisk immediately. Add the flax meal, and cinnamon. Stir to combine. Remove from heat, add lucuma powder and serve immediately.

Topping suggestions: sliced strawberries, blueberries or few almonds.

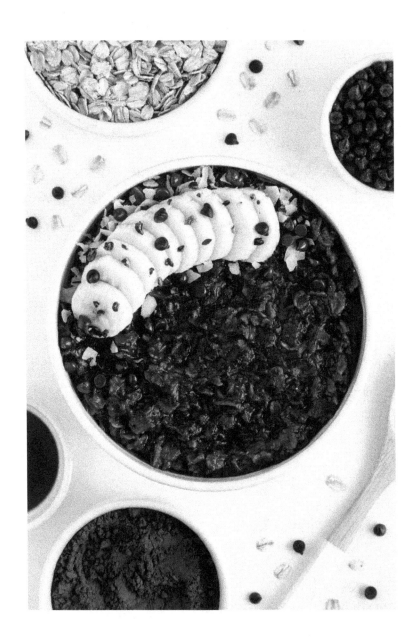

Flax and Blueberry Vanilla Overnight Oats

Ingredients - Allergies: SF, GF, EF, V, NF

    1/2 cup dry oats

    1/3 cup water

    1/2 cup low-fat yogurt

    1/2 tsp. ground vanilla bean

    2 tbsp. flax seeds meal A pinch of salt

    Blueberries, almonds, blackberries, lucuma powder for topping

Instructions

Add the ingredients (except for toppings) to the bowl in the evening. Refrigerate overnight.

In the morning, stir up the mixture. It should be thick. Add the toppings of your choice.

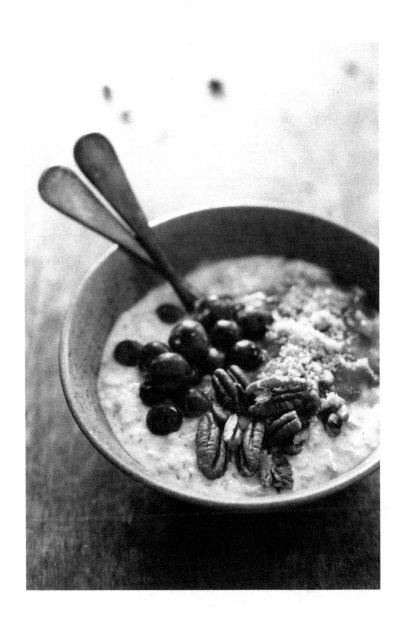

Apple Oatmeal

Ingredients - Allergies: SF, GF, DF, EF, V, NF
   1/2 grated apple
   1/2 cup dry oats
   1 cups water
   Dash of cinnamon
   1 tsp. lucuma powder

   Instructions
Cook the oats with the water for 3-5 minutes.
Add grated apple and cinnamon. Stir in the lucuma powder.

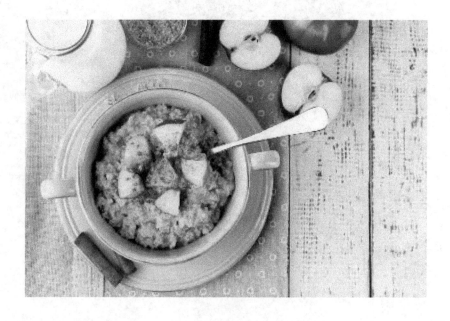

Coconut Pomegranate Oatmeal

Ingredients - Allergies: SF, GF, DF, EF, V, NF

- 1/2 cup dry oats
- 1/3 cup coconut milk
- 1 cups water
- 2 tbs. shredded unsweetened coconut
- 1 tbs. flax seeds meal
- 1 tbs. lucuma powder
- 4 tbs. pomegranateseeds

Instructions

Cook oats with the coconut milk, water, and salt.

Stir in the coconut, lucuma powder and flaxseed meal.

Sprinkle withextra coconut and pomegranate seeds.

SAVORY BREAKFASTS

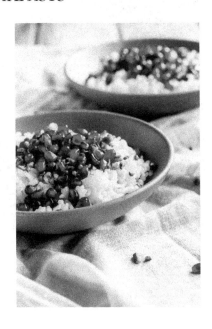

Egg pizza crust

Ingredients - Allergies: SF, GF, DF, NF

2 eggs

1/4 cup of coconut flour

1/2 cup of coconut milk

1 small crushed garlic clove

Mix and make an omelet.

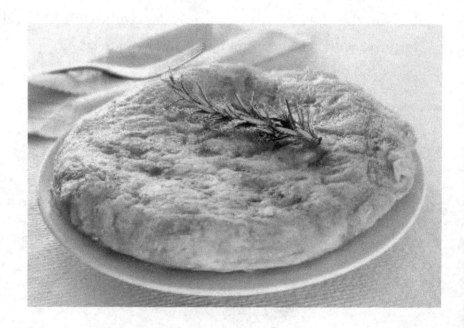

Egg Muffins

Ingredients - Allergies: SF, GF, DF, NF
Serving: 4 muffins

  4 eggs
   1/2 cup diced green bell pepper
   1/2 cup diced onion
   1/2 cup spinach
   1/4 tsp. salt
   1/8 tsp. ground black pepper
   2 tbsp. water

Instructions

Heat the oven to 350 degrees F. Oil 4 muffin cups. Beat eggs together. Mix in bell pepper, spinach, onion, salt, black pepper, and water. Pour the mixture into muffin cups. Bake in the oven until muffins are done in the middle.

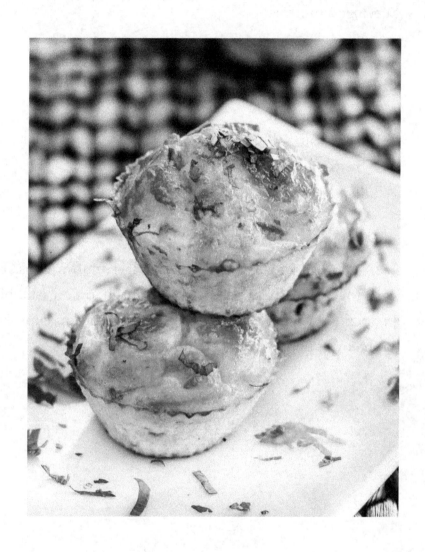

Smoked Salmon Scrambled Eggs

Ingredients - Allergies: SF, GF, DF, NF

1 tsp coconut oil

2 eggs

1 Tbs water

2 oz smoked salmon, sliced

1/4 avocado

ground black pepper, to taste

2 chives, minced (or use 1 green onion, thinly sliced)

Instructions

Heat a skillet over medium heat. Add coconut oil to pan when hot. Meanwhile, scramble eggs. Add eggs to the hot skillet, along with smoked salmon. Stirring continuously, cook eggs until soft and fluffy. Remove from heat. Top with avocado, black pepper, and chives to serve.

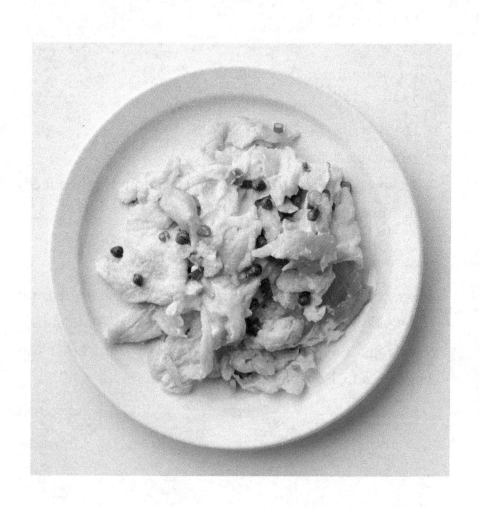

Egg Bake

Ingredients - Allergies: SF, GF, DF, NF

1/2 cup chopped red peppers or spinach
1/4 cup zucchini
1/2 tbsp. coconut oil
1/4 cup sliced green onions
2 eggs
1/4 cup coconut milk
1/8 cup almond flour
1 tbsp. minced fresh parsley
1/4 tsp. dried basil
1/8 tsp. salt
1/8 tsp. ground black pepper

Instructions

Preheat oven to 350 degrees F. Put coconut oil in a skillet. Heat it to medium heat. Add mushrooms, onions, zucchini and red pepper (or spinach) until vegetables are tender, about 5 minutes. Drain veggies and spread them over the baking dish.

Beat eggs in a bowl with milk, flour, parsley, basil, salt, and pepper. Pour egg mixture into baking dish.

Bake in preheated oven until the center is set (approx. 35 to 40 minutes).

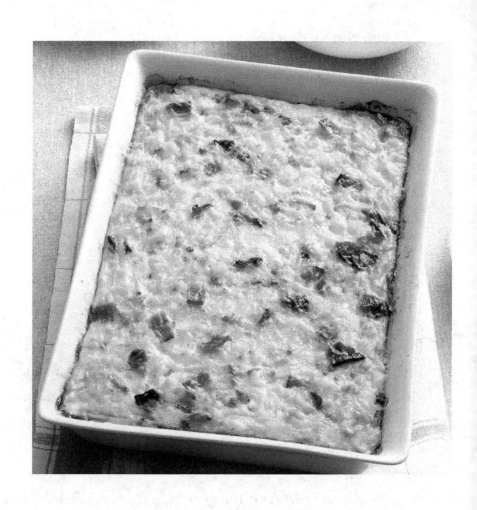

Frittata

Ingredients - Allergies: SF, GF, DF, NF

1 tbsp. olive oil or avocado oil
1/2 Zucchini, sliced
1/4 cup torn freshspinach
1 tbsp. sliced green onions
1/4 tsp. crushed garlic, salt and pepper to taste
1/8 cup coconut milk
2 eggs

Instructions

Heat olive oil in a skillet over medium heat. Add zucchini and cook until tender. Mix in spinach, green onions, and garlic. Season with salt and pepper. Continue cooking until spinach is wilted.

In a separate bowl, beat together eggs and coconut milk. Pour into the skillet over the vegetables. Reduce heat to low, cover, and cook until eggs are firm (5 to7 minutes).

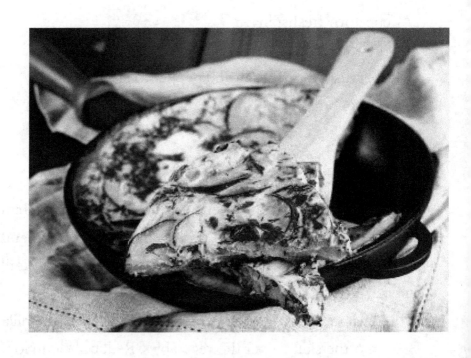

Superfoods Naan Pancakes Crepes

Ingredients - Allergies: SF, GF, DF, EF, V
> 1/2 cup almond flour
> 1/2 cup Tapioca Flour
> 1 cup Coconut Milk
> Salt, coconut oil

Instructions

Mix all the ingredients together.

Heat a pan over medium heat and pour batter to desired thickness. Once thebatter looks firm, flip it over to cook the other side.

If you want this to be a dessert crepe or pancake, then omit the salt. You can addminced garlic or ginger in the batter if you want, or some spices.

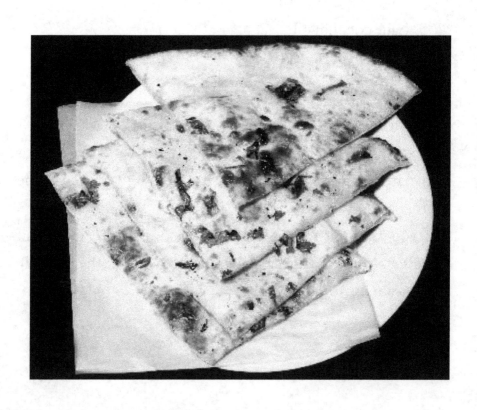

Zucchini Pancakes

Ingredients - Allergies: SF, GF, DF

    1 small zucchini

    1 tbsp. chopped onion

    2 beaten eggs

    3 tbsp. almond flour

    1/2 tsp. salt

    1/2 tsp. ground black pepper

    coconut oil

Instructions

Heat the oven to 300 degrees F.

Grate the zucchini into a bowl and stir in the onion and eggs.
Stir in 6 tbsp. of the flour, salt, and pepper.

Heat a large sauté pan over medium heat and add coconut oil in the pan. When the oil is hot, lower the heat to medium-low and add batter into the pan. Cook the pancakes about 2 minutes on each side, until browned. Place the pancakes inthe oven.

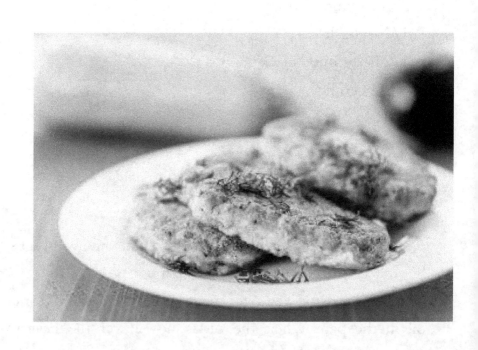

Put the liquid in first. Surrounded by tea or yogurt, the blender blades can move freely. Next, add chunks of fruits or vegetables. Leafy greens are going into the pitcher last. Preferred liquid is green tea, but you can use almond or coconut milk or herbal tea.

Start slow. If your blender has speeds, start it on low to break up big pieces of fruit. Continue blending until you get a puree. If your blender can pulse, pulse a few times before switching to a puree mode. Once you have your liquid and fruit pureed, start adding greens, very slowly. Wait until previous batch of greens has been completely blended.

Thicken? Added too much tea or coconut milk? Thicken your smoothie by adding ice cubes, flax meal, chia seeds or oatmeal. Once you get used to various tastes of smoothies, add any seaweed, spirulina, chlorella powder or ginger for additional kick. Experiment with any Superfoods in powder form at this point. Think of adding any nut butter or sesame paste too or some Superfoods oils.

Rotate! Rotate your greens; don't always drink the same smoothie! At the beginning try 2 different greens every week and later introduce third and fourth one weekly. And keep rotating them. Don't use spinach and kale all the time.

Try beets greens, they have a pinch of pink in them and

that add great color to your smoothie. Here is the list of leafy green for you to try: spinach, kale, dandelion, chards, beet leaves, arugula, lettuce, collard greens, bok choy, cabbage, cilantro, parsley.

Flavor! Flavor smoothies with ground vanilla bean, cinnamon, lucuma powder, nutmeg, cloves, almond butter, cayenne pepper, ginger or just about any seeds or chopped nuts combination.

Not only are green smoothies high in nutrients, vitamins and fiber, they can also make any vegetable you probably don't like (be it kale, spinach or broccoli) taste great. The secret behind blending the perfect smoothie is using sweet fruits or nuts or seeds to give your drink a unique taste.

There's a reason kale and spinach seem to be the main ingredients in almost every green smoothie. Not only do they give smoothies their verdant color, they are also packed with calcium, protein and iron.

Although blending alone increases the accessibility of carotenoids, since the presence of fats is known to increase carotenoid absorption from leafy greens, it is possible that coconut oil, nuts and seeds in a smoothie could increase absorption further.

If you can't find some ingredient, replace it with the closest one.

GREEN SMOOTHIES

Zucchini Apples Smoothie

- 1/2 cup zucchini
- 1 Apple
- 3/4 avocado
- 1 stalk Celery
- 1 Lemon
- 1 tbsp. Spirulina
- 1 1/2 cups crushed ice

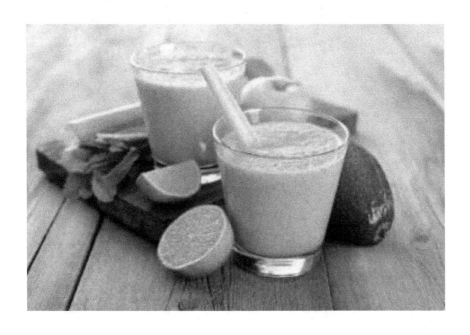

Dandelion Smoothie

1 cup Dandelion greens

1 cup Spinach

½ cup tahini

1 Red Radish

1 tbsp. <u>chia</u> seeds

1 cup lavender tea

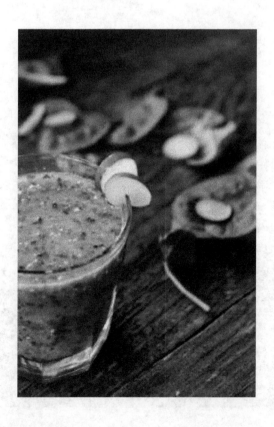

Broccoli Apple Smoothie

1 Apple

1 cup Broccoli

1 tbsp. Cilantro

1 Celery stalk

1 cup crushed ice

1 tbsp. crushed Seaweed

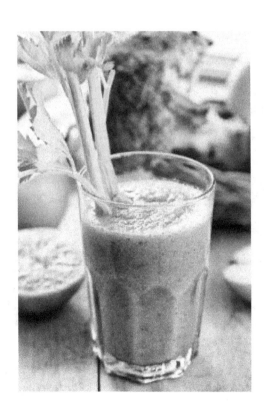

Salad Smoothie

1 cup spinach

½ cucumber

1/2 small onion

2 tablespoons Parsley

2 tablespoons lemon juice

1 cup crushed ice

1 tbsp. <u>olive</u> oil or <u>cumin</u> oil

¼ cup Wheatgrass

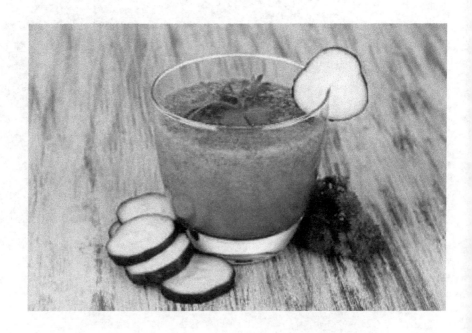

Avocado Kale Smoothie

1 cup Kale

½ Avocado

1 cup Cucumber

1 Celery Stalk

1 tbsp. chia seeds

1 cup chamomile tea

1 tbsp. Spirulina

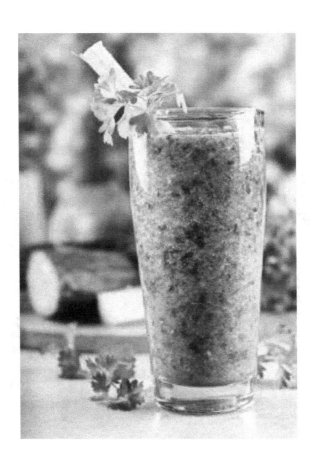

Watercress Smoothie

1 cup Watercress

½ cup <u>almond</u> butter

2 small cucumbers

1 cup coconut milk

1 tbsp. Chlorella

1 tbsp. Black cumin seeds – sprinkle on top and garnish with parsley

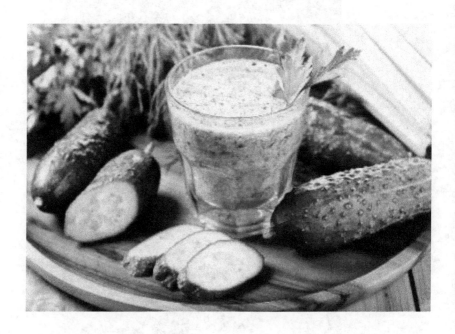

Beet Greens Smoothie

1 cup Beet Greens

2 tbsp. Pumpkin seeds butter

1 cup Strawberry

1 tbsp. Sesame seeds

1 tbsp. hemp seeds

1 cup chamomile tea

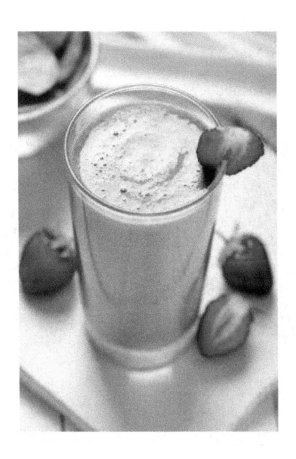

Broccoli Leeks Cucumber smoothie

1 cup Broccoli

2 tbsp. Cashew butter

2 Leeks

2 Cucumbers

1 Lime

½ cup Lettuce

½ cup Leaf Lettuce

1 tbsp. Matcha

1 cup crushed ice

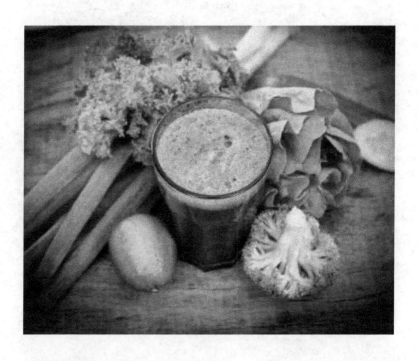

Cacao Spinach Smoothie

2 cups spinach

1 cup blueberries, frozen

1 tablespoons dark cocoa powder

½ cup unsweetened almond milk

1/2 cup crushed ice

1 tsp lucuma powder

1 tbsp. Matcha powder

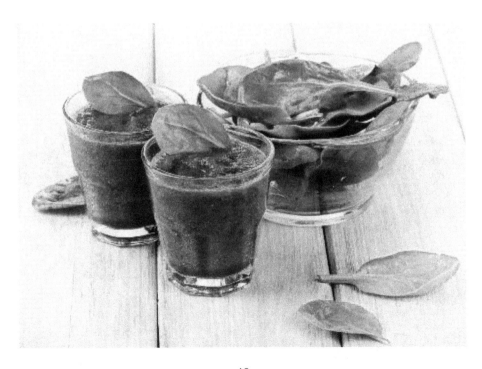

Flax Almond Butter Smoothie

½ cup plain yogurt

2 tablespoons <u>almond</u> butter

2 cups spinach

3 strawberries

1/2 cup crushed ice

1 teaspoon <u>flax</u> seeds

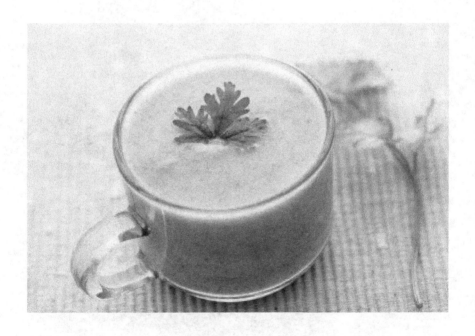

Apple Kale Smoothie

1 cup kale

½ cup coconut milk

1 tbsp. Maca

¼ teaspoon cinnamon

1 Apple

Pinch of nutmeg

1 clove

3 ice cubes

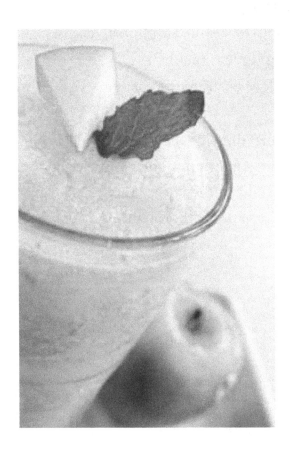

Large Fiber Loaded Salad as a meal on its own

Allergies: SF, GF, EF, NF

This is what I eat every second evening and I can't get enough of it!!! This is the real secret to lose weight while having full stomach with grade.

Ingredients!!
   2 cup of spinach
   2 cup of shredded cabbage
   Yogurt dressing
   Cayenne pepper (optional)
   Few sprigs of cilantro (optional)
   3 spring (green) onions
   10 o.z. low-fat farmers' cheese

Pour yogurt dressing into the salad bowl. Add farmers' cheese and mix thoroughly. Cut spring onions in small pieces and add to the cheese mixture and mix. Add spinach and cabbage and mix thoroughly. Add spices (optional).

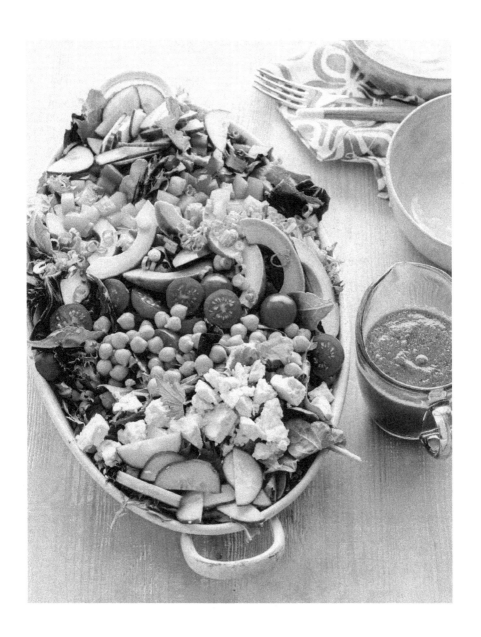

Greek Salad

Allergies: SF, GF, EF, NF
  1 head romaine lettuce
  1/2 lb. plump tomatoes
  3 oz. Greek or black olives, sliced
  2 oz. sliced radishes
  4 oz. low-fat feta or goat cheese
  2 oz. anchovies (optional)

Dressing:
  2 oz. olive oil or avocado oil
  2 oz. fresh lemon juice
  1/2 tsp. dried oregano
  1/4 tsp. black pepper
  1/4 tsp. salt
  2 cloves garlic, minced

Wash and cut lettuce into pieces. Slice tomatoes in quarters. Combine olives, lettuce, tomatoes, and radishes in large bowl. Mix dressing ingredients together and toss with vegetables. Pour out into a shallow serving bowl. Crumble feta/goat cheese over all, and arrange anchovy fillets on top (if desired).

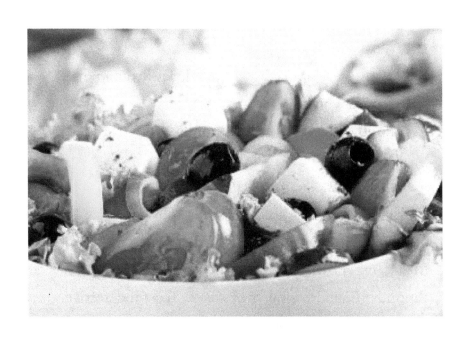

Strawberry Spinach Salad

Ingredients - Allergies: SF, GF, DF, EF, V

- 1 tbsp. black sesame seeds
- 1 tbsp. poppy seeds
- 1/4 cup <u>olive</u> oil or <u>cumin</u> oil
- 1/8 cup lemon juice
- 1/8 tsp. paprika
- 1/2 bag fresh spinach - chopped, washed and dried
- 1 cup strawberries, sliced
- 1/4 cup toasted slivered almonds

Instructions

Whisk together the sesame seeds, olive oil, poppy seeds, paprika, lemon juice and onion. Refrigerate.

In a large bowl, combine the spinach, strawberries and almonds. Pour dressing over salad. Toss and refrigerate 15 minutes before serving.

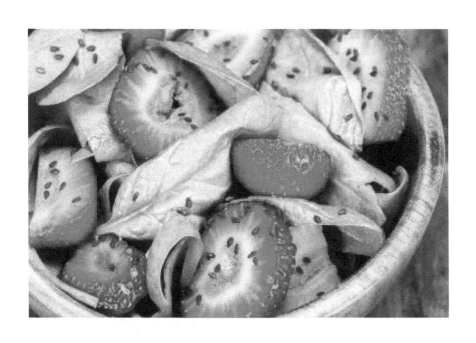

Greek Cucumber Salad

Ingredients - Allergies: SF, GF, EF, NF
  2 cucumbers, sliced
  1 teaspoon salt
  2 tbsp. lemon juice
  1/4 tsp. paprika
  1/4 tsp. white pepper
  1/2 clove garlic, minced
  2 fresh green onions, diced
  1 cup thick Greek Yogurt
  1/4 tsp. paprika Instructions

Slice cucumbers thinly, sprinkle with salt and mix. Set aside for one hour. Mix lemon juice, water, garlic, paprika and white pepper, and set aside. Squeeze liquid from cucumber slices a few at a time, and place slices in the bowl. Discard liquid. Add lemon juice mixture, green onions, and yogurt. Mix and sprinkle additional paprika or dill over top. Chill for 1-2 hours.

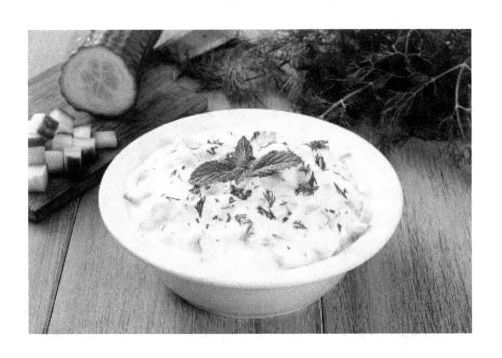

Mediterranean Salad

Ingredients - Allergies: SF, GF, DF, EF, V, NF

- 1 small head romaine lettuce, torn
- 1 tomato, diced
- 1 small cucumber, sliced
- 1/2 green bell pepper, sliced
- 1/2 small onion, cut into rings
- 3 radishes, thinly sliced
- 1/4 cup flat leaf parsley, chopped
- 1/4 cup <u>olive</u> oil or <u>avocado</u> oil
- 2 tbsp. lemon juice
- 1 garlic clove, minced
- Salt & pepper
- 1 tsp. fresh mint, minced

Instructions

Combine lettuce, tomatoes, cucumber, pepper, onion, radishes & parsley in a salad bowl. Whisk together olive oil, lemon juice, garlic, salt, pepper & mint. Pour over salad & toss to coat.

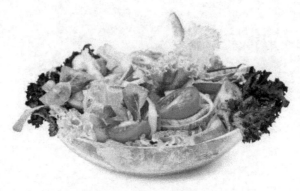

Pomegranate Avocado salad

Ingredients - Allergies: SF, GF, DF, EF, V

  2 cups mixed greens, spinach, arugula, red leaf lettuce

  1 ripeavocado, cut into 1/2-inch pieces

  1 cup pomegranate seeds

  1/2 cup pecan

  1/2 cup blackberries

  1/2 cup cherry tomatoes

  Olive oil, salt, lemon juice

Instructions

Combine greens, pecan, cut avocado, tomatoes, pomegranates and blackberries in a salad bowl. Whisk together salt, olive oil and lemonjuice and pour over salad.

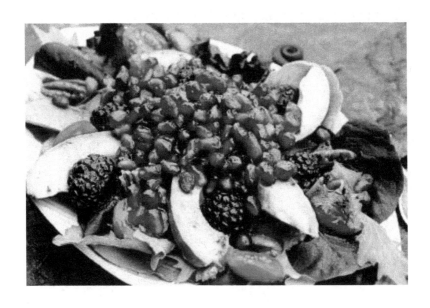

Apple Coleslaw

Ingredients - Allergies: SF, GF, DF, EF, V, NF

    2 cups chopped cabbage (various color)

    1 tart apple chopped

    1 celery, chopped

    1 red pepper chopped

    4 tsp. olive oil or avocado oil

    juice of 1 lemon

    1 Tbs. lucuma powder (optional)

    dash sea salt

Instructions

Toss the cabbage, apple, celery, and pepper together in a large bowl. In a smaller bowl, whisk remaining ingredients. Drizzle over coleslaw and toss to coat.

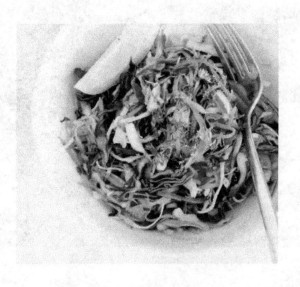

Hummus

Ingredients - Allergies: SF, GF, DF, EF, V, NF
1/2 cup cooked chickpeas (garbanzo beans)
1/2 small lemon
2 Tbsp. tahini
Half of a garlic clove, minced
1 tbsp. olive oil or cumin oil, plus more for serving
1/2 tsp. salt
1/4 tsp. ground cumin
2 to 3 tbsp. water
Dash of ground paprika for serving

Instructions
Combine tahini and lemon juice and blend for 1 minute. Add the olive oil, minced garlic, cumin and the salt to tahini and lemon mixture. Process for 30seconds, scrape sides and then process 30 seconds more.

Add half of the chickpeas to the food processor and process for 1 minute. Scrape sides, add remaining chickpeas and process for 1 to 2 minutes.

Transfer the hummus into a bowl then drizzle about 1 tbsp. of olive oil over thetop and sprinkle with paprika.

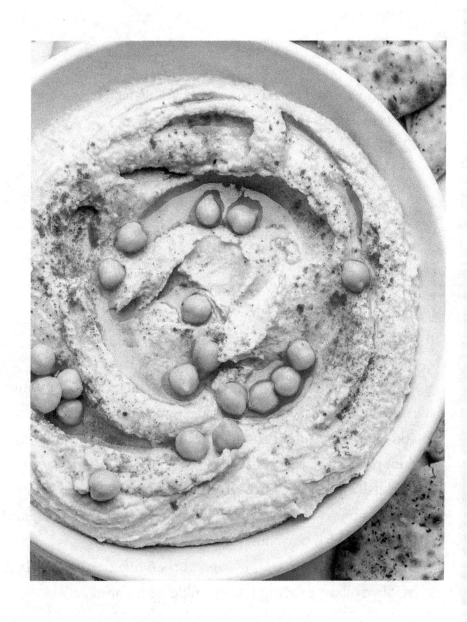

Guacamole

Ingredients - Allergies: SF, GF, DF, EF, V, NF

2 ripe avocados

2 tbsp. freshly squeezed lemon juice (1 lemon)

4 dashes hot pepper sauce

1/4 cup diced onion

1 garlic clove, minced

1/2 tsp. salt

1/2 tsp. ground black pepper

1 small tomato, seeded, and small-diced

Instructions

Cut the avocados in half, remove the pits, and scoop the flesh out. Immediately add the lemon juice, hot pepper sauce, garlic, onion, salt, and pepper and toss well. Dice avocados. Add the tomatoes. Mix well and taste for salt and pepper.

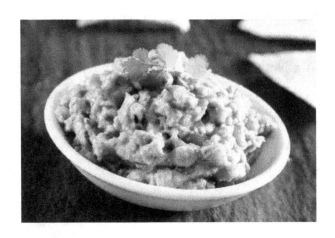

BABAGANOUSH

Ingredients - Allergies: SF, GF, DF, EF, V, NF

1 eggplant
1/4 cup tahini, plus more as needed
1 garlic clove, minced
1/8 cup fresh lemon juice, plus more as needed
1pinch ground cumin
salt, to taste
1 tbsp. extra-virgin <u>olive</u> oil or <u>avocado</u> oil
1 tbsp. chopped flat-leaf parsley
1/4 cup brine-cured black olives, such as Kalamata

Instructions:
Grill eggplantfor 10 to 15 minutes. Heat the oven (375 F).
Put the eggplant to a baking sheet and bake 15-20 minutes or
until very soft.Remove from the oven, let cool, and peel off
and discard the skin. Put the eggplant flesh in a bowl. Using
a fork, mash the eggplant to a paste.
Add the 1/4 cup tahini, garlic, cumin, 1/4 cup lemon juice
and mix well. Seasonwith salt to taste. Transfer the mixture
to a serving bowl and spread with the back of a spoon to
form a shallow well. Drizzle the olive oil over the top and
sprinkle with the parsley.
Serve at room temperature.

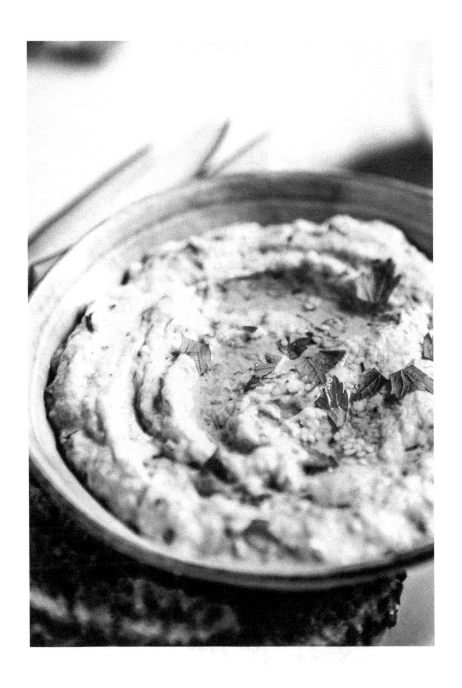

Espinacas a la Catalana

Ingredients - Allergies: SF, GF, DF, EF, V

1 cup spinach

1 cloves garlic

2 tbsp cashews

<u>olive</u> oil or <u>avocado</u> oil

Instructions

Wash the spinach and trim off the stems. Steam the spinach for few minutes.

Peel and slice the garlic. Pour a few tablespoons of olive oil and cover the bottom of a frying pan. Heat pan on medium and sauté garlic for 1-2 minutes. Add the cashews to the pan and continue to sauté for 1 minute. Add the spinachand mix well, coating with oil. Salt to taste.

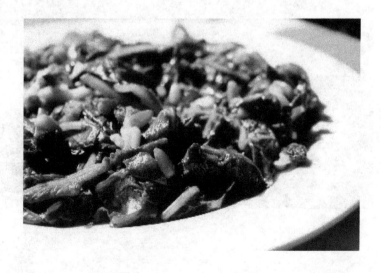

Tapenade

Ingredients - Allergies: SF, GF, DF, EF, V, NF

1/4 pound olives with pit removed

2 anchovy fillets, rinsed

1 small clove garlic, minced

2 tbsp. capers

2 fresh basil leaves

1 tbsp. freshly squeezed lemon juice

1 tbsp. extra-virgin olive oil or cumin oil

Instructions

Rinse the olives in cool water. Place all ingredients in the bowl of a food processor. Process to combine, until it becomes a coarse paste. Transfer to abowl and serve.

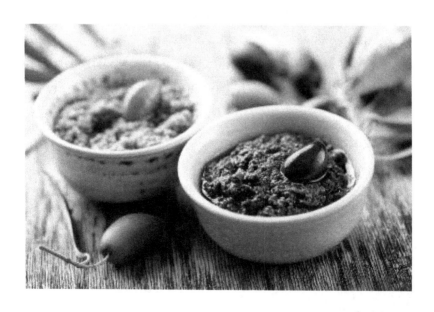

Red Pepper Dip

Ingredients - Allergies: SF, GF, EF, NF
  1/2 pound red peppers
  1/2 cup farmers' cheese
  1 Tbsp. virgin <u>olive</u> oil or <u>avocado</u> oil
  1/2 tbsp minced garlic
  Lemon juice, salt, basil, oregano, red pepper flakes to taste.

Instructions

Roast the peppers. Cover them and cool for about 15 minutes. Peel the peppers and remove the seeds and stems. Chop the peppers.

Transfer the peppers and garlic to a food processor and process until smooth. Add the farmers' cheese and garlic and process until smooth. With the machine running, add olive oil and lemon juice. Add the basil, oregano, red pepper flakes, and 1/8 tsp. salt, and process until smooth. Adjust the seasoning, to taste. Pour to a bowl and refrigerate.

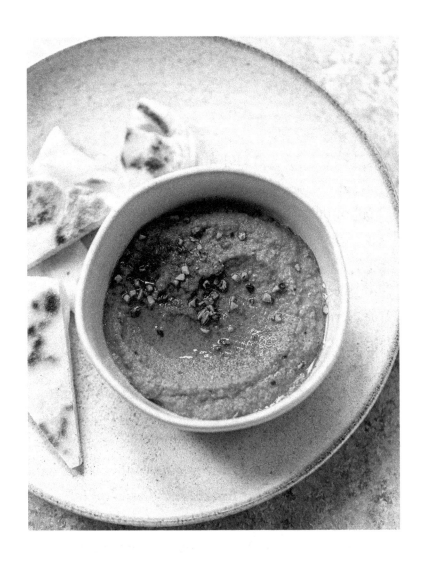

Caponata

Ingredients - Allergies: SF, GF, DF

Coconut oil
1 large eggplants, cut into large chunks
1 tsp. dried oregano
Sea salt
Freshly ground black pepper
1 small onion, peeled and finely chopped
1 clove garlic, peeled and finely sliced
1 small bunch fresh flat-leaf parsley, leaves picked and stalks finely chopped
1 tbsp. salted capers, rinsed, soaked and drained
1 handful green olives, stones removed
2 tbsp. lemon juice
2 large ripe tomatoes, roughly chopped
coconut oil
2 tbsp. slivered almonds, lightly toasted, optional

Instructions

Heat coconut oil in a pan and add eggplant, oregano and salt. Cook on a highheat for around 4 or 5 minutes. Add the onion, garlic and parsley stalks and continue cooking for another few minutes. Add drained capers and the olives and lemon juice. When all the juice has evaporated, add the tomatoes and simmer until tender.

Season with salt and olive oil to taste before serving. Sprinkle with almonds.

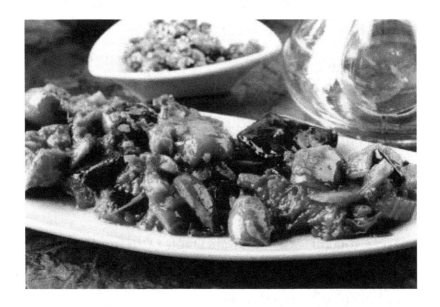

Cream of Broccoli Soup

Ingredients - Allergies: SF, GF, EF, NF
   1 pound broccoli, fresh
   1 cup water
   1/4 tsp. salt, pepper to taste
   1/4 cup tapioca flour, mixed with 1 cup cold water
   1/4 cup coconut cream
   1/4 cup low-fat farmers' cheese Steam or boil broccoli until it gets tender.

Instructions
Put 1 cup of water and coconut cream in top of double boiler. Add salt, cheese and pepper. Heat until cheese gets melted.
Add broccoli. Mix water and tapioca flour in a small bowl.
Stir tapioca mixture into cheese mixture in double boiler and heatuntil soup thickens.

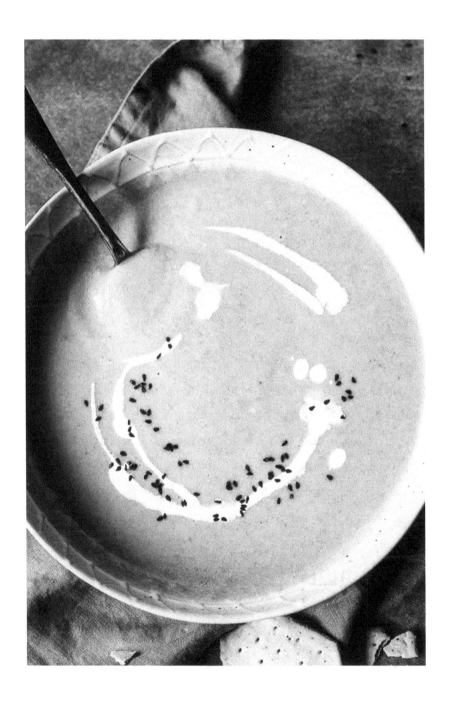

Lentil Soup

Ingredients - Allergies: SF, GF, DF, EF, NF
- 1 tbsp. olive oil or avocado oil
- 1/2 cup finely chopped onion
- 1/4 cup chopped carrot
- 1/4 cup chopped celery
- 1 teaspoons salt
- 1/2 pound lentils
- 1/2 cup chopped tomatoes
- 1 quart chicken or vegetable broth
- 1/4 tsp. ground coriander & toasted cumin

Instructions

Place the olive oil into a large Dutch oven. Set over medium heat. Once hot, add the celery, onion, carrot and salt and do until the onions are translucent. Add the lentils, tomatoes, cumin, broth and coriander and stir to combine. Increase the heat and bring just to a boil. Reduce the heat, cover and simmer at a low until the lentils are tender (approx. 35 to 40 minutes). Puree with a bender to your preferred consistency (optional). Serve immediately.

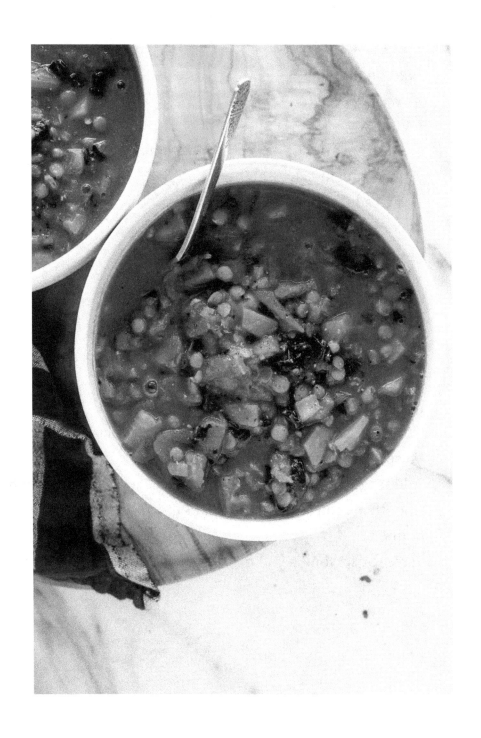

Cold CucumberAvocado Soup

Ingredients
Allergies: SF, GF, EF, NF

1 cucumber peeled, seeded and cut into
2-inch chunks
1 avocado, peeled
1 chopped scallions
1 cup chicken broth
1/3 cup Greek low-fat yogurt
1 tbsp. lemon juice
1/4 tsp. ground pepper, or to tasteGarnish:
Chopped chives, dill, mint, scallions or cucumber

Instructions
Combine the cucumber, avocado and scallions in a blender. Pulseuntil chopped.
Add yogurt, broth and lemon juice and continue until smooth.Season with pepper and salt to taste and chill for 4 hours.
Taste for seasoning and garnish.

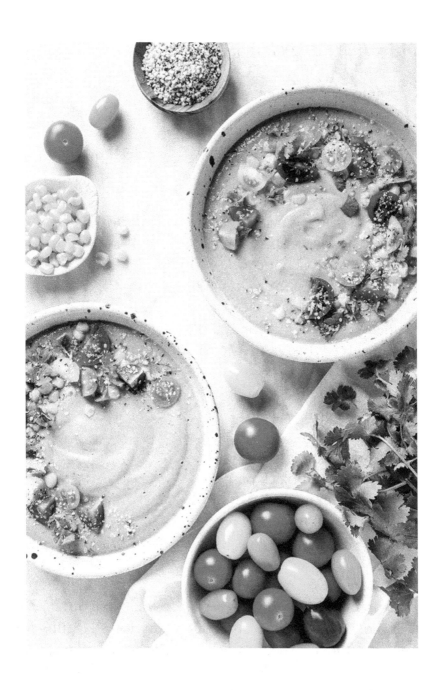

Bouillabaisse

Ingredients - Allergies: SF, GF, DF, EF, NF

1 pound of 3 different kinds of fish fillets
1/4 cup Coconut oil
1 pounds of Oysters, clams, or mussels
1/3 cup cooked shrimp, crab, or lobster meat, or rock lobster tails
1/3 cup thinly sliced onions
1 Shallot or the white parts of 1 leek, thinly sliced
1 cloves garlic,crushed
1 small tomato, chopped
1/2 sweet red pepper, chopped
2 stalks celery, thinly sliced
1-inch slice of fennel or 1/2 tsp. of fennel seed
1 sprigs fresh thyme or 1/4 tsp. dried thyme
1 bay leaf
1 whole cloves
Zest of half an orange
1/4 tsp. saffron
1 teaspoons salt
1/4 tsp. ground black pepper
1/3 cup clam juice or fish broth
1 Tbps lemon juice
1/3 cup white wine

Instructions

In a large saucepan heat 1/8 cup of the coconut oil. When it is hot, add onions and shallots (or leeks). Sauté for a minute. Add crushed garlic, and sweet red pepper. Add celery, tomato, and fennel. Stir the vegetables until well coated. Add another 1/8 cup of coconut oil, bay leaf, thyme, cloves and the orange zest. Cook until the onion is golden. Cut fish fillets into 2-inch pieces. Add 1 cup of water and the pieces of fish to the vegetable mixture. Bring to a boil, then reduce heat and let it simmer, uncovered, for about 10 minutes. Add clams, oysters or mussels (optional) and crabmeat, shrimp or lobster tails, cut into pieces. Add salt, saffron and pepper. Add lemon juice, clam juice, and white wine. Bring to a simmer again and cook for 5 minutes longer.

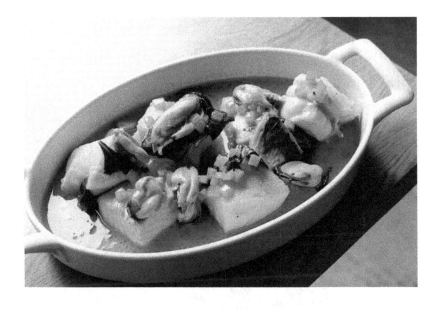

Gaspacho

Ingredients - Allergies: SF, GF, DF, EF, V, NF
  1/4 cup of <u>flax</u> seeds meal
  1 pound tomatoes, diced
  1 red pepper or 1 green pepper, diced
  1 small cucumber, peeled and diced
  1 cloves of garlic, peeled and crushed
  ¼ cup extra virgin <u>olive</u> oil or <u>cumin</u> oil
  1 tbsp. lemon juice
  Salt, to taste

Instructions

Mix the peppers, tomatoes and cucumber with the crushed garlic and olive oil in the bowl of a blender. Add flax meal to the mixture. Blend until smooth. Add salt and lemon juice to taste and stir well.

Refrigerate. Serve with black olives, hard-boiled egg, cilantro, mint orparsley.

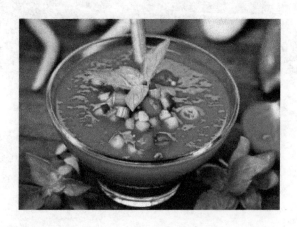

Italian Beef Soup

Ingredients - Allergies: SF, GF, DF, EF, NF
1/3 pound minced beef
1 clove garlic, minced
1 cups beef broth
1 large tomato
1/2 cup sliced carrots
1/2 cup cooked beans
1 small zucchini, cubed
1 cups spinach - rinsed and torn
1/8 tsp. black pepper
1/8 tsp. salt Brown beef with garlic in a stockpot.

Instructions
Stir in broth, carrots and tomatoes. Season with salt and pepper. Reduce heat, cover, and simmer for 15minutes.
Stir in beans with liquid and zucchini. Cover, and simmer until zucchini is tender. Remove from heat, add spinach and cover. Serve after 5minutes.

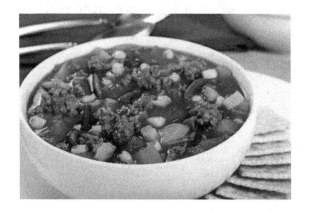

Creamy roasted mushroom

Ingredients - Allergies: SF, GF, DF, EF, V, NF

- 1/2 pound Portobello mushrooms, cut into 1inch pieces •
- 1/4 pound shiitakemushrooms, stemmed
- 2 tbsp. olive oil or avocado oil • 1 cups vegetable broth
- 1 tbsp. coconut oil
- 1/2 onion, chopped
- 1 garlic cloves, minced
- 1 tbsp. arrowroot flour
- 1/4 cup coconut cream
- 1/4 tsp. chopped thyme

Instructions

Heat oven to 400°F. Line one large baking sheets with foil. Spread mushrooms and drizzle some olive oil on them. Season with salt and pepper and toss. Cover with foil and bake them for half an hour. Uncover and continue baking 15 minutes more. Cool slightly. Mix one half of the mushrooms with one can of broth in a blender. Set aside.

Melt coconut oil in a large pot over high heat. Add onion and garlic and sauté until onion is translucent. Add flour and stir 2 minutes. Add cream, broth, and thyme. Stir in remaining cooked mushrooms and mushroom puree. Simmer overlow heat until thickened (approx. 10 minutes). Season to taste with salt and pepper.

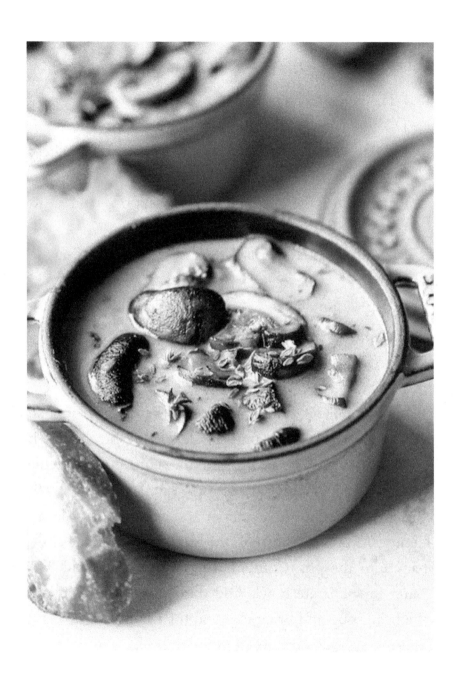

Black Bean Soup

Ingredients - Allergies: SF, GF, DF, EF, NF

1 Tbsp. cup Coconut Oil

1/4 cup Onion, Diced

1/4 cup Carrots, Diced

1/4 cup Green Bell Pepper, Diced

1 cup beef broth

1 pound cooked Black Beans

1 tbsp. lemon juice

1 teaspoons chopped

Garlic

1 teaspoons Salt

1/4 tsp. Black Pepper, Ground

1 teaspoons Chili Powder

4 oz. pork

1 tbsp. tapioca flour

2 tbsp. Water

Instructions

Place coconut oil, onion, carrot, and bell pepper in a stock pot. Cook the veggies until tender. Bring broth to a boil. Add cooked beans, broth and the remaining ingredients (except tapioca flour and 2 tbsp. water) to the vegetables. Bring that mixture to a simmer and cook approximately 15 minutes. Puree 1 quart of the soup in a blender and put back into the pot. Combine the tapioca flour and 2 tbsp. water in a separate bowl. Add the tapioca flour mixture to the bean soup and bring to a boil for 1 minute.

Kale White Bean Pork Soup

Ingredients - Allergies: SF, GF, DF, EF, NF

1 tbsp. each extra-virgin olive oil and <u>coconut oil</u>
1 tbsp. chili powder
1/2 tbsp. jalapeno hot sauce
1/2 pound bone-in pork chops
Salt
2 stalks celery, chopped
1 small white onion, chopped
1 cloves garlic, chopped
1 cup chicken broth
1 cups diced tomatoes
1/2 cup cooked white beans
2 cups packed Kale *Instructions*

Preheat the broiler. Whisk hot sauce, 1 tbsp. olive oil and a pinch of chili powder in a bowl. Season the pork chops with 1/2 tsp. salt. Rub chops with the spice mixture on both sides and place them on a rack set over a baking sheet. Set aside.

Heat 1 tbsp. coconut oil in a large pot over high heat. Add the celery, garlic, onion and the remaining chili powder. Cook until onions are translucent, stirring (approx. 8 minutes).

Add tomatoes and the chicken broth to the pot. Cook and stir occasionally until reduced by about one-third (approx. 7

minutes). Add the kale and the beans.

Reduce the heat to medium, cover and cook until the kale is tender (approx. 7minutes). Add up to 1/2 cup water if the mixture looks dry and season with salt.

In the meantime, broil the pork until browned (approx. 4 to 6 minutes). Flip and broil until cooked through. Serve with the kale and beans.

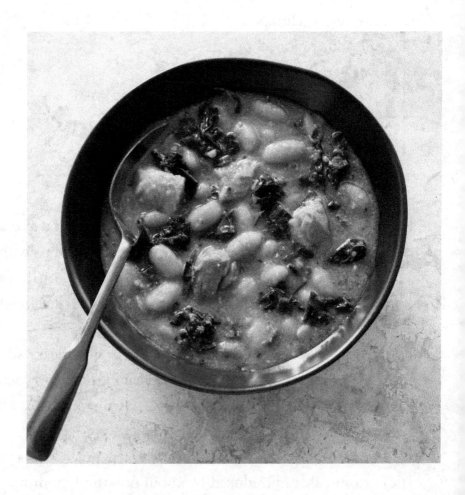

Ingredients - Allergies: SF, GF, DF, NF

2 cups quarts chicken broth

1 tbsps. Tapioca flour, mixed in 1/4 cup cold water

2 eggs, slightly beaten with a fork

2 scallions, chopped, including green ends

Instructions

Bring broth to a boil. Slowly pour in the tapioca flour mixture while stirring the broth. The broth should thicken. Reduce heat
and let it simmer. Mix in the eggs very slowly while stirring. As soon as the last drop of egg is in, turn off the heat. Serve with chopped scallions on top.

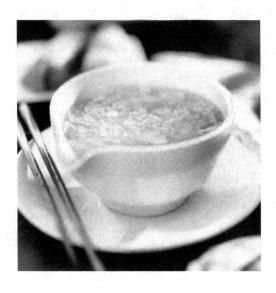

Creamy Tomato Basil Soup

Ingredients - Allergies: SF, GF, DF, EF, V, NF

2 tomatoes - peeled, seeded and diced

2 cups tomato juice*

5 leaves fresh basil

1/2 cup coconut cream

salt to taste

ground black pepper to taste *Instructions*

Combine tomatoes and tomato juice in stock pot. Simmer 30 minutes. Puree mixture with basil leaves in a processor. Put back in a stock pot and add coconut cream. Add salt and pepper to taste.

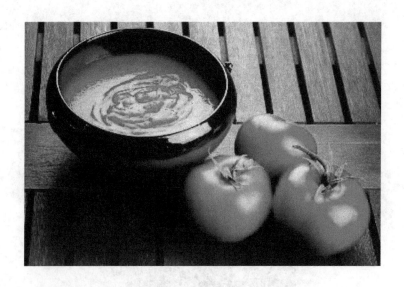

Minestrone

Ingredients - Allergies: SF, GF, DF, EF, NF

1 tbsp. coconut oil

1 cloves garlic, chopped

1/2 onions, chopped

1/2 cups chopped celery

2 carrots, sliced

1 cup chicken broth

1/2 cups water

1 cup tomato sauce

1/2 oz. red wine (optional)

1/2 cup cooked kidney beans

1/2 cups green beans

1/2 cups baby spinach, rinsed

1 small zucchinis, quartered and sliced

1/2 tbsp. chopped oregano

1 tbsp. chopped basil

salt and pepper to taste

1/2 tbsp. <u>olive</u> oil or <u>cumin</u> oil *Instructions*

Heat coconut oil over medium heat in a stock pot, and sauté garlic for few minutes. Add onion and sauté for few more minutes. Add celery and carrots and sauté for 2 minutes.

Add chicken broth, tomato sauce and water and bring to boil, stirring frequently. Add red wine at this point. Reduce heat to low and add kidney beans, zucchini, green beans, spinach leaves, oregano, basil, salt and pepper. Simmer for 30 to 40 minutes.

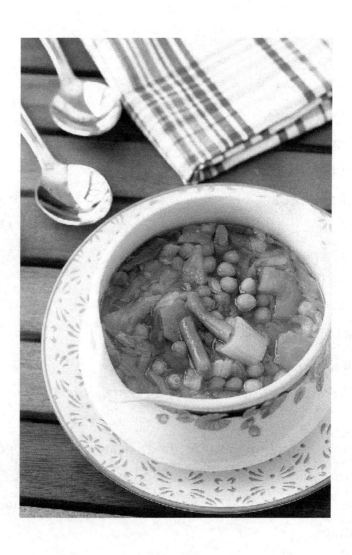

Grilled Meats & Salad

Caribbean Chicken salad

Ingredients - Allergies: SF, GF, DF, EF, NF

2 boneless skinless chicken breasts *Marinade*
1/2 cup fish sauce
2 tomatoes (seeded and chopped)
1/2 cup chopped onion
2 tsps. jalapeno chilies (minced)
2 tsps. chopped cilantro fresh

Lucuma powder Lime Dressing:
1/4 cup mustard
1/4 cup lucuma powder
1 tbsp coconut oil
1 1/2 tbsps. lemon juice
1 1/2 tsps. lime juice
3/4 lb mixed greens

Instructions

Blend all the marinade ingredients in a small bowl with a hand blender. Cover and chill. Marinate the chicken for at least two hours in the fridge. Grill the chicken for few minutes per side or until done.

Serve the greens into 2 large salad bowls. Slice the chicken into thin strips. Divide among bowls. Pour the dressing aside and serve with the salads.

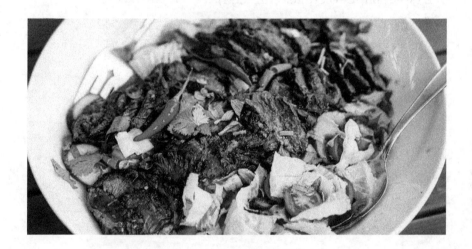

Herb Crusted Salmon

Allergies: SF, GF, DF, EF, NF

Rub some tarragon, chives and parsley over 2 salmon steaks and add some salt and pepper. Heat the pan with 1 tsp of coconut oil to medium high and place the salmon, skin-side up in the pan. Cook until golden brown on 1 side, about 4 minutes. Turn the fish over and cook until it feels firm to the touch. Salmon is done when it flakes easily with a fork. Serve with a wedge of lemon.

Large mixed spinach and lettuce salad with "Italian Dressing" and some thyme sprinkled on top of it. Salad can be as large as you want, but use the prescribed amount of the dressing.

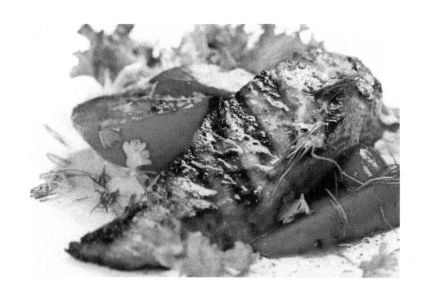

Stews, Chilies and Curries

Vegetarian Chili

Ingredients - Allergies: SF, GF, DF, EF, V, NF

1 tbsp. coconut oil
1/2 cup chopped onions
1/2 cup chopped carrots
1 cloves garlic, minced
1/2 cup chopped green bell pepper
1/2 cup chopped red bell pepper
1/4 cup chopped celery
1/2 tbsp. chili powder
1/2 cups chopped mushrooms
1 cup chopped tomatoes
1 cups cooked kidney beans
1/2 tbsp. ground cumin
1/2 teaspoons oregano
1/2 teaspoons crushed basil leaves

Instructions

Heat coconut oil in a large saucepan and add onions, carrots and garlic; sauté until tender. Stir in green pepper, red pepper, celery andchili powder.
Cook, stirring often, until vegetables are tender, about 6 minutes.
To the vegetables add mushrooms; cook 4 minutes. Stir in tomatoes, kidney beans, corn, cumin, oregano and basil. Bring to a boil. Reduce heat to medium. Cover and simmer for 20 minutes, stirring occasionally.

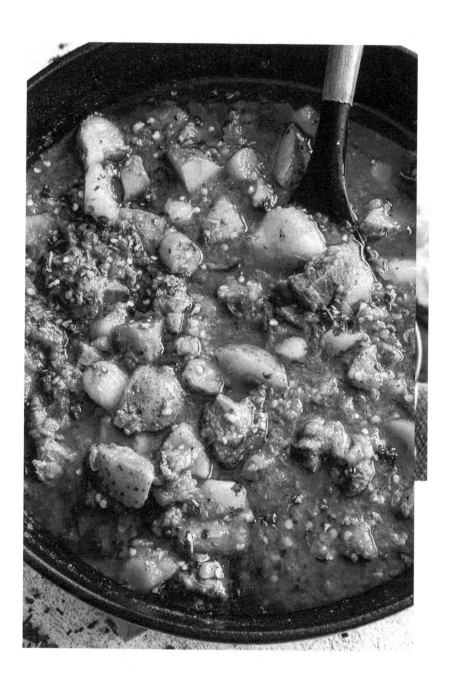

White Chicken Chili

Ingredients - Allergies: SF, GF, DF, EF, NF

2 large boneless, skinless chicken breasts
1 green bell peppers
1/2 yellow onion
1/2 jalapeno
1/4 cup diced green chilies (optional)
1/4 cup of spring onions
1 tbsp. coconut oil
1/2 cup cooked white beans
2 cups chicken or vegetable broth
1/2 tsp. ground cumin
1/8 tsp. cayenne pepper
salt to taste

Instructions

Bring a pot of water to boil. Add the chicken breasts and cook until cooked through. Drain water and allow chicken to cool. When cool,shred and set aside.

Dice the bell peppers, jalapeno and onion. Melt the coconut oil in a pot over high heat. Add the peppers and onions and sauté until soft,approx. 8-10 minutes.

Add the broth, beans, chicken and spices to the pot. Stir and bring to a low boil. Cover and simmer for 25-30 minutes.

Simmer for 10 more minutes and stir occasionally. Remove from heat. Let stand for 10 minutes to thicken. Top with cilantro.

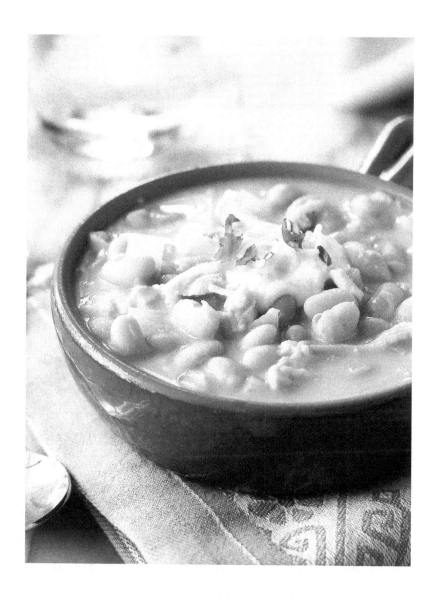

Kale Pork

Ingredients - Allergies: SF, GF, DF, EF, NF

1 tbsp. <u>coconut oil</u>
1/2 pound pork tenderloin, trimmed and cut into 1-inch pieces • 1/4 tsp. salt
1/2 medium onion, finely chopped
2 cloves garlic, minced
1 teaspoons paprika
1/8 tsp. crushed red pepper (optional)
1/2 cup white wine
2 plump tomatoes, chopped
2 cups chicken broth
1/2 bunch kale, chopped
1 cups cooked white beans

Instructions

Heat oil in a pot over medium heat. Add pork, season with salt and cook until no longer pink. Transfer to a plate and leave juices in the pot.

Add onion to the pot and cook until turns translucent. Add paprika, garlic and crushed red pepper and cook about 30 seconds. Add tomatoes and wine, increase heat and stir to scrape up any browned bits. Add broth. Bring to a boil.

Add kale and stir until it wilts. Lower the heat and simmer, until the kale is tender. Stir in beans, pork and pork juices. Simmer for 2 more minutes.

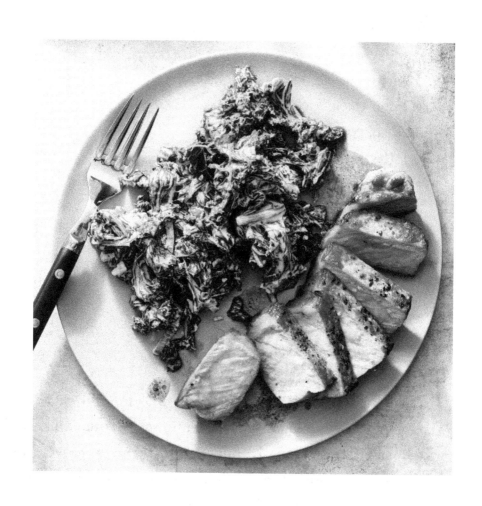

30. Minute Squash Cauliflower and Green Peppers Coconut Curry

Ingredients - Allergies: SF, GF, DF, EF, V, NF

Curry Paste

1 cups peeled, chopped squash

1 cup thick coconut milk

1 tbsp. coconut oil

1 tbsp. lucuma powder

1 pound tomatoes

1/2 cup brown rice, uncooked

1/2 cup choppedCauliflower

1/2 cup chopped Green Peppers

Cilantro for topping

Instructions

Cook brown rice. Set aside.

Make Curry Paste. Pour the coconut milk into the skillet and mix the curry andlucuma powder into the coconut milk. Add the cauliflower, squash, and green peppers. Cover and simmer until squash is tender. Remove from heat and let stand for 10 minutes. The sauce will thicken.

Serve the curry with chopped cilantro.

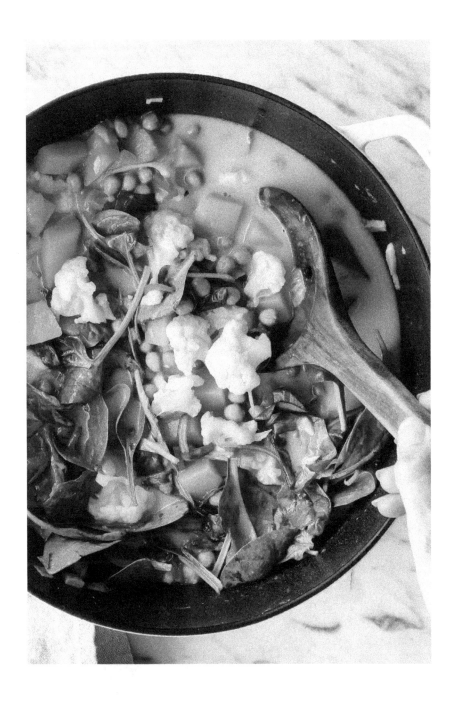

CPSIA information can be obtained
at www.ICGtesting.com
Printed in the USA
BVHW090851140621
609525BV00002B/55

9 781458 355034